Where Do Babies Come From?

Margaret Sheffield

Illustrated by Sheila Bewley

Jonathan Cape Thirty Bedford Square London

Everybody in the world started life as a baby, like the baby in this picture, which is drinking milk from one of its mother's breasts.

Everybody was a baby once, and every baby is made in the same way, by two grown-up people, a man and a woman – the baby's mother and father.

There is no way of coming into the world fully grown.

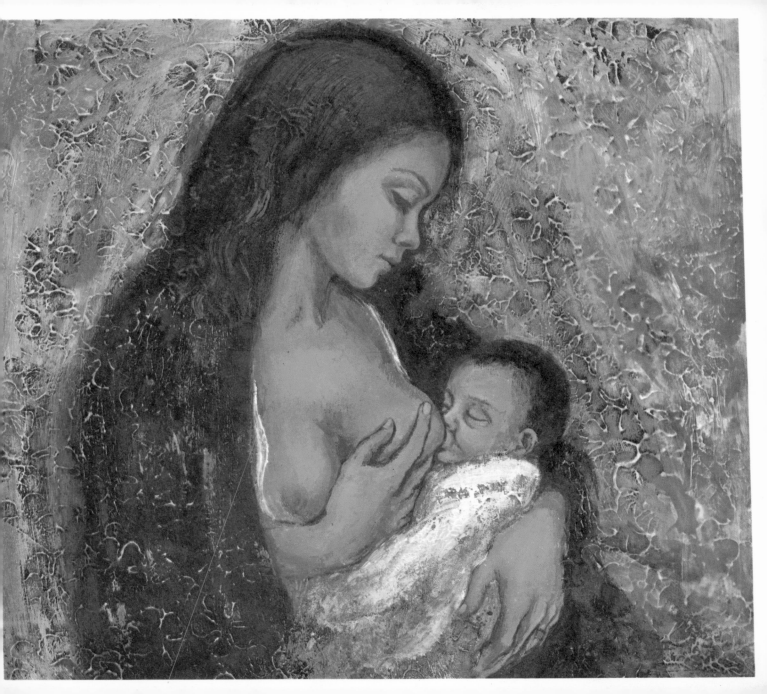

Babies begin life inside their mothers' bodies, in a special place called the womb.

You can't see the womb, because it is right inside the mother's body. But you can easily tell when a woman is going to have a baby because her whole belly looks bigger and rounder.

The woman in the picture is going to have a baby. She is pregnant.

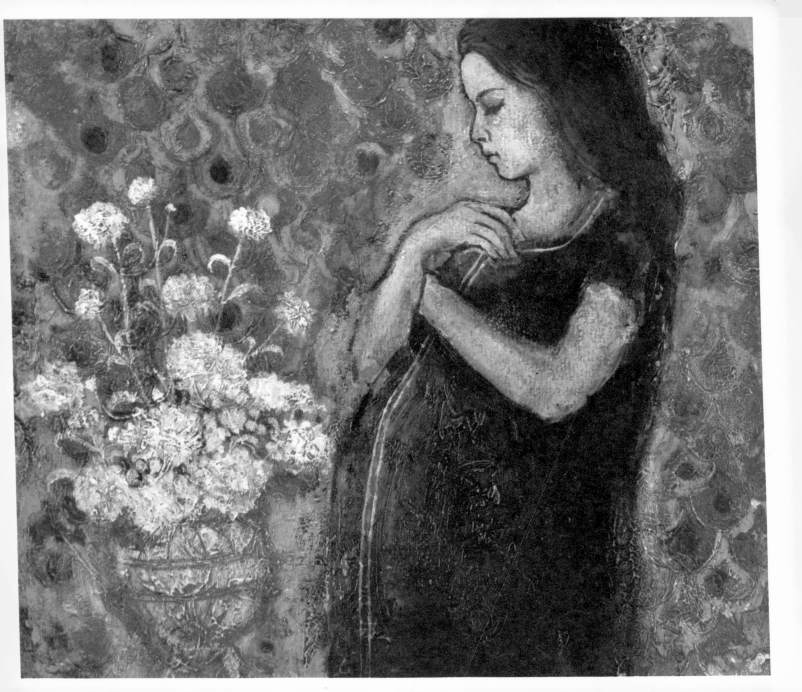

If you could look inside the body of a pregnant woman you would see the unborn baby curled up inside the womb where it is safe and warm and protected from the outside world. The womb is kept tightly closed until the day the baby is ready to be born.

The way out of the womb is through the vagina, which ends in an opening between the woman's legs. The opening is covered by two flaps of soft skin, like lips, so that from the outside the end of the vagina looks like a slit, where these two flaps of skin come together and form a line. Grown-up women have curly hair growing around this part (on the front, and on the outside only).

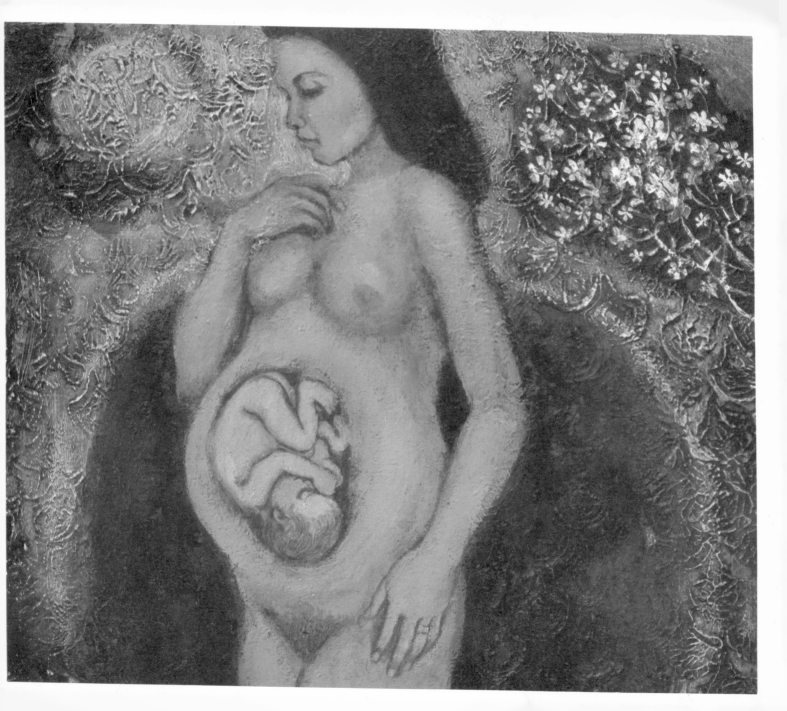

Young girls have a womb and a vagina but they can't have babies until the womb is fully developed and their bodies are working like a grown-up woman's body.

Young girls also don't have any breasts or any hair under their arms or around the end of the vagina. These things come as they grow up.

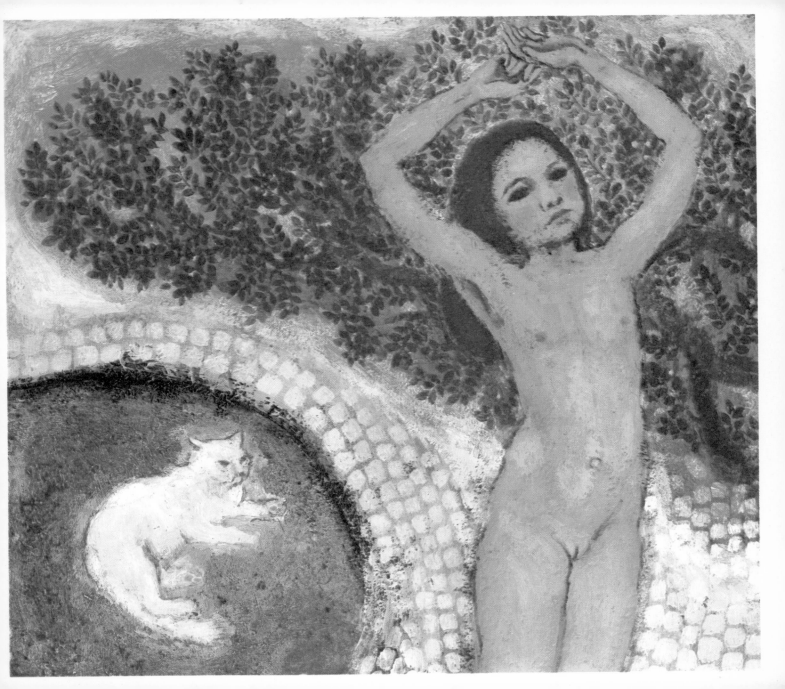

Boys are different from girls, of course.

Boys have a penis, which is joined to the body between their legs. Under the penis there is a small bag of skin with two small round-shaped things inside. The name for these is testicles, although because they're round like balls many people just call them balls.

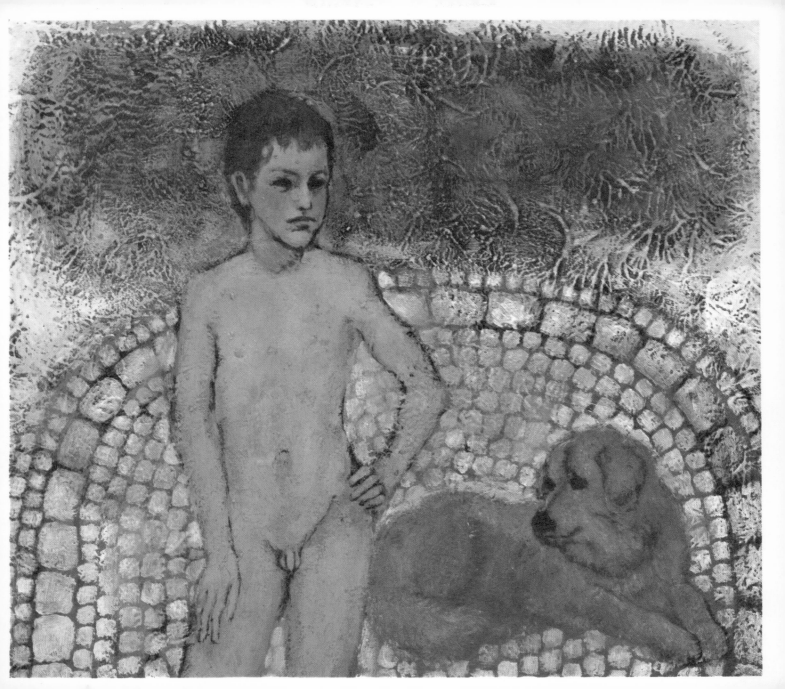

Men look like boys except that they're bigger and they have hair growing on various parts of their bodies.

Grown-up men have a special liquid in their testicles which comes out through the penis – not urine, which also comes out through the penis, but a special, different liquid with things called sperms in it. Sperms are invisible; you can only see them with a microscope.

A sperm is what makes a baby grow inside a woman.

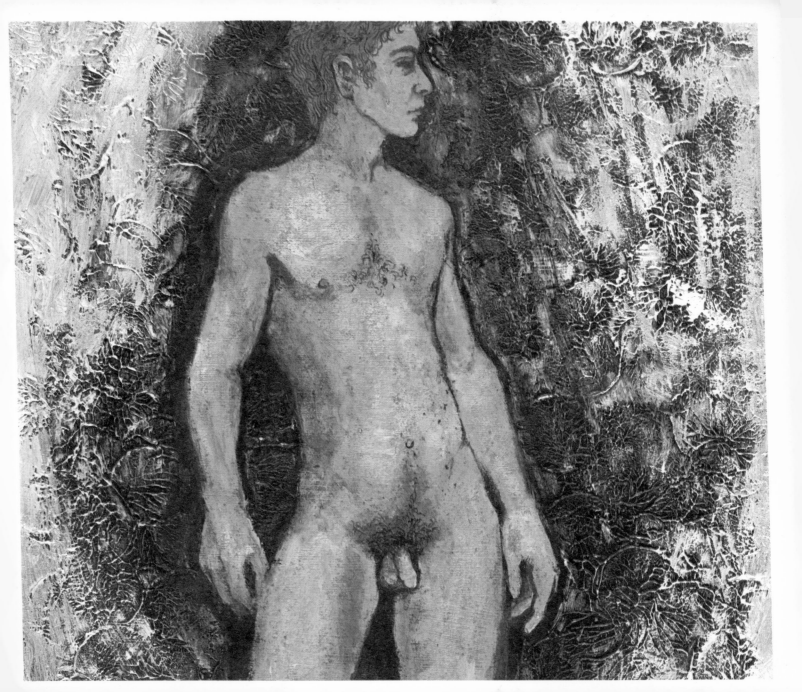

Women have eggs in their bodies, tiny eggs about the size of these dots ... They're kept right inside the woman's body, near the womb.

To make a baby, a sperm from the man has to get to one of these eggs in the woman.

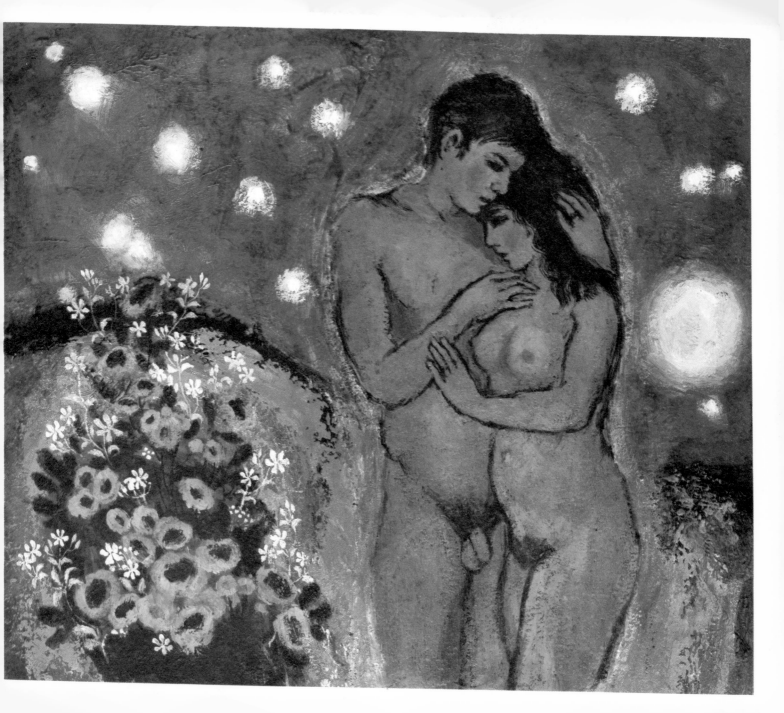

The only way for the sperm to get to an egg is through the woman's vagina.

This is how babies are begun, with the man lying so close to the woman that his penis can fit into her vagina.

If one of his sperms can get to one of her eggs, a baby will begin to grow.

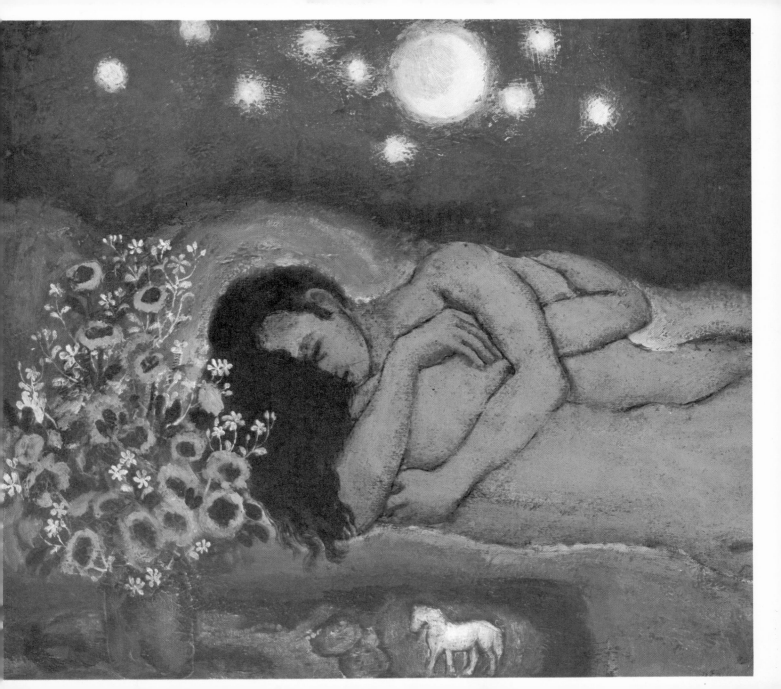

If a sperm manages to join up with an egg they begin to grow into a baby. But the egg is so small to begin with that it takes three months to grow to the size shown in the picture. That's what a real baby looks like after it has been growing in the womb for about three months. It weighs about one ounce. It is about four inches long.

But although it is so tiny it is already beginning to get the shape of a person, with a head and arms and legs.

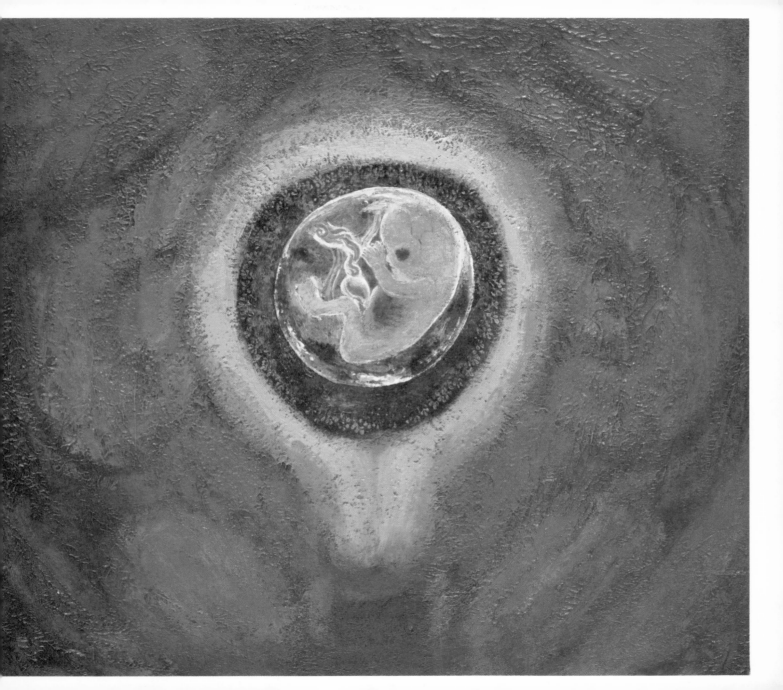

After the baby has been growing for six months it looks much more like a person. It can kick its feet and move its arms about. It has eyelashes and hair and fingernails. It has a heart that beats. Its food and oxygen are carried to it by blood that passes through the cord joining the baby's body to the inside of the womb. You can see the cord in the picture.

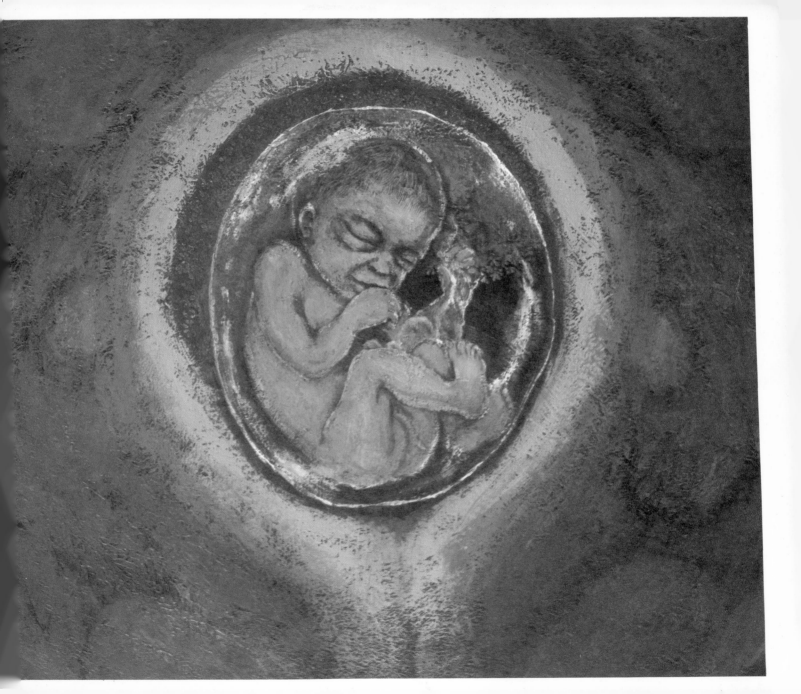

After nine months inside the womb the baby is
ready to be born. It has everything a new baby
should have. It's probably about twenty inches
long and between five and ten pounds in weight. In
the month before it is born it usually settles down
low in the womb, upside down, ready to come out.

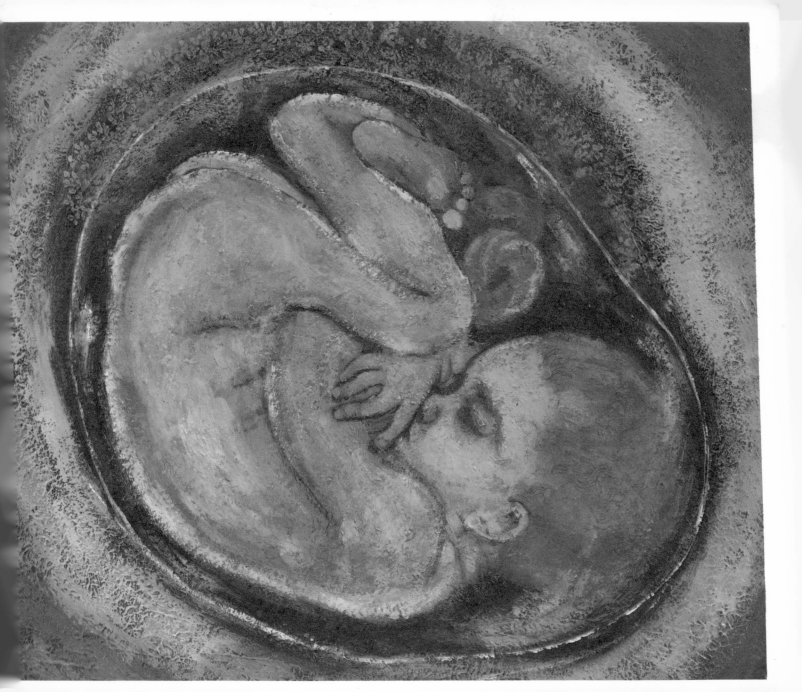

To be born the baby has to come out of the womb and down through the vagina. Mothers usually have a doctor or a nurse to help them with the birth, because it can take hours and hours, sometimes more than a day. The muscles that held the womb tightly shut for nine months gradually relax, and other muscles in the mother's body push the baby out.

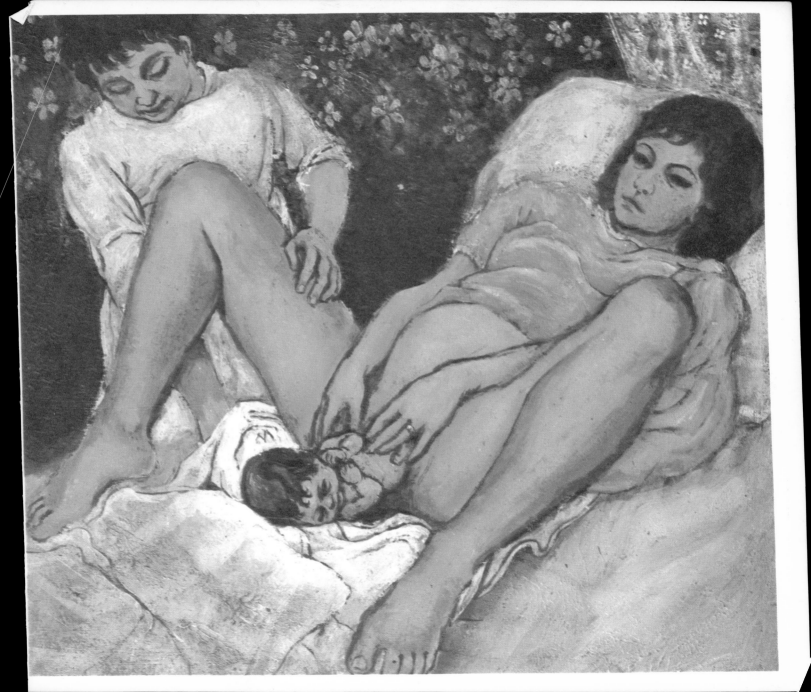

When the baby is born it still has the cord that joined it to the inside of the womb. The nurse ties pieces of tape on the cord, to stop the blood coming out, and then cuts it, because it isn't needed any more. This doesn't hurt either the mother or the baby. Neither of them can feel it happening.

After this has been done the baby really is a separate person.

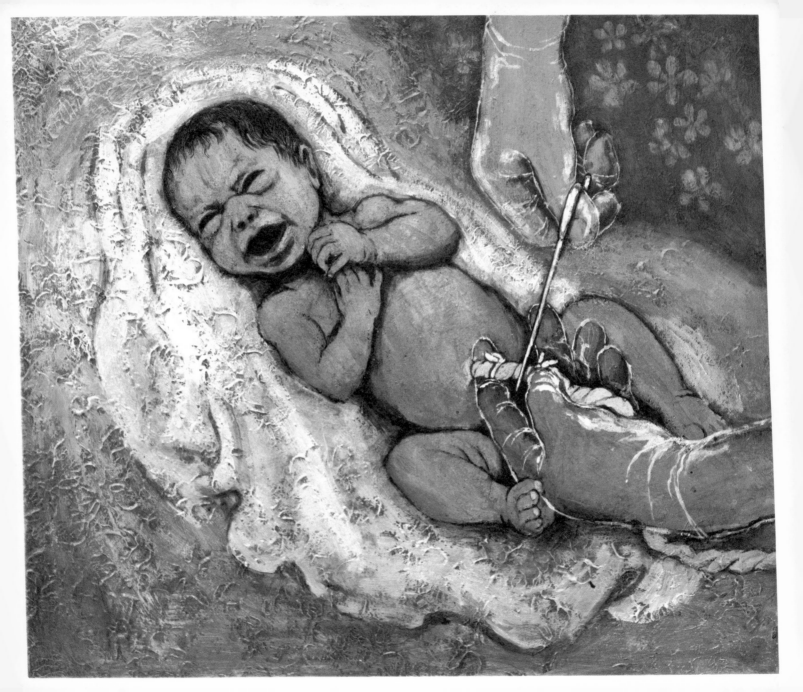

This is a boy baby. He has a penis. It's impossible to tell whether a baby is a boy or a girl while it is still in the womb. But as soon as it is born the doctor looks to see whether it has a penis or a vagina and immediately says to the mother, 'It's a boy!' or, 'It's a girl!'

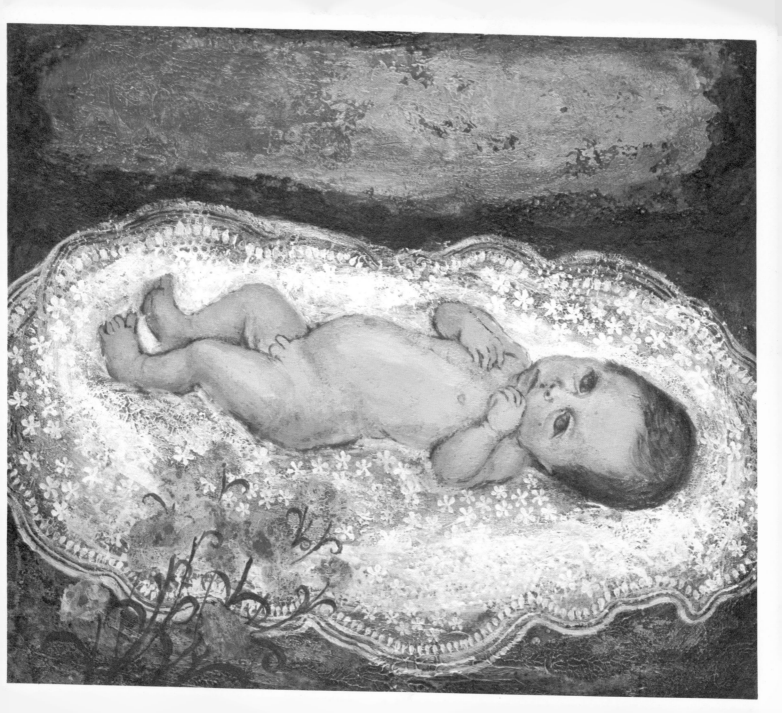

This is a girl baby. She has a vagina. Inside she has a tiny womb – and when she grows up she may have a baby herself.

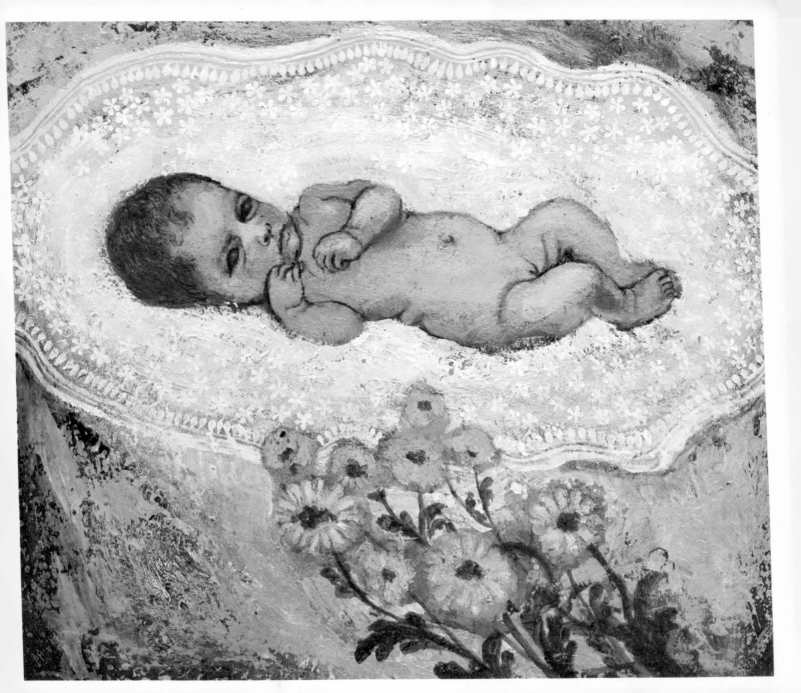

Everybody in the world started life as a baby and was made in the same way, by a man and a woman together. Everybody grew first inside their mother's womb and then was born.

And that's where babies come from.

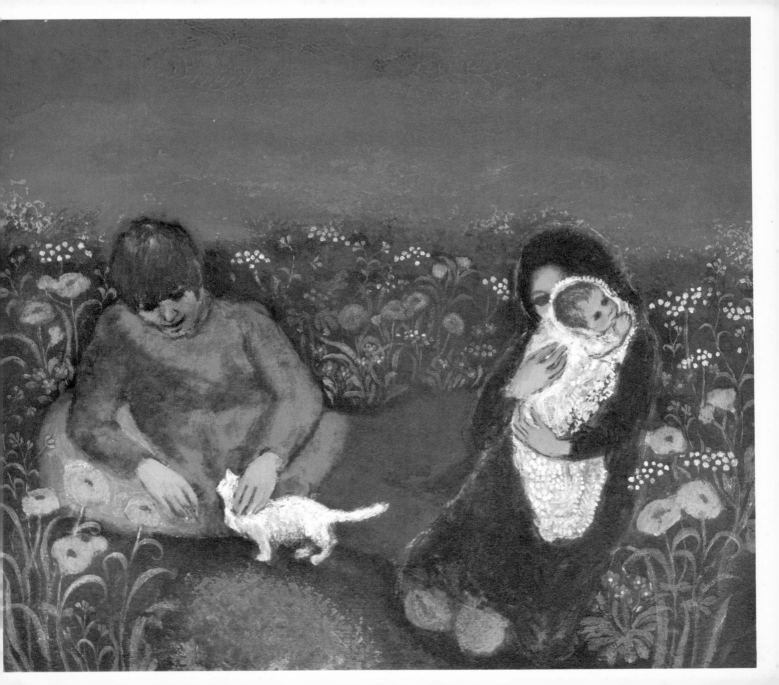

First published 1973
Reprinted 1974, 1975, 1976, 1978
© 1972 by Sheila Bewley and Margaret Sheffield

Jonathan Cape Ltd, 30 Bedford Square, London WC1

ISBN Hardback 0 224 00717 3
      Paperback 0 224 00732 7

Printed in Great Britain by Sackville Press Billericay Ltd.